HEALING

Arise!

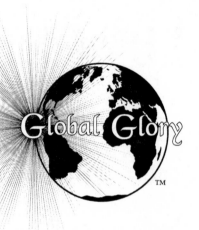

GLOBAL GLORY®
PRESENTS:

HEALING

Arise!

JAN TMEIZEH

Healing Arise
by Jan Tmeizeh

Published by:

Global Glory
P.O. Box 310
Oliver Springs, TN 37840 USA

Visit our website: www.globalglory.gg

Cover design by Lynn Alessandra Bacarella Wright and Saifiel Tmeizeh.

Typesetting by Ruel Tmeizeh.

ISBN 978-0-9850955-7-4
ISBN 978-0-9850955-8-1 (electronic)

Library of Congress Control Number: 2012944627

Printed in the United States of America
First Edition, August 2012

10 9 8 7 6 5 4 3 2 1

Why so many translations?

When one is familiar with certain translations, the Scriptures can go "in one ear and out the other." I desire the words to stop in the brain, be meditated upon, and flow into the heart.

I make no claim that every jot and tittle of this book is either literarily or grammatically correct. There are instances in which I knowingly disregarded convention. It is not a formal work, so I took liberty with the rules. Some capitalization, or the lack thereof, and the manner in which certain statements were phrased are examples.

With the faith, prayers, and hard work of Lynn Alessandra Bacarella Wright, Ruel Tmeizeh, and Saifiel Tmeizeh, I was able to get this book into print to share.

They would say, and I say with them, "All glory to the Lord!"

This book is dedicated to Yeshua, to them, and to you, the reader.

"Let's *live* Jani!

—at least until we find out if He wants us to or not!"

Lynn Alessandra Bacarella Wright

(see page 40)

Contents

Preface and Introduction xiii

Firm Foundation 1

Translated 13

Faith 19

Removing Hindrances 31

Counterattack 43

Resurrection Life 49

Faith Action 107

Destiny Arise 111

Preface and Introduction

A WORD FROM JAN:

I know that there are probably thousands of books on healing available, but what I wanted to offer in these pages is a small book, easy to carry around with you; something like a handy handbook.

If you read these instructions carefully, you will discover not only how to obtain your healing, but also how to keep and maintain your healing. Moreover, you will learn why some fail to receive healing, or fail to keep it after they have been healed.

The Bible is a book of God's commands *and* His promises. However, we cannot expect to receive the promises without fulfilling the prerequisites of the commands.

The Bible is not like any other book. It is the most precious item; the greatest thing to be had. It is the most valuable possession you can ever own. Why would I make such an incredible statement? Because through the Bible you can obtain everything you will ever need.

This remarkable book is like a box of seeds. All seeds are life–giving. Inherent in the DNA of a seed are all the properties necessary to bring life after its kind. Isaiah 55:11 (NLT) reads, *It is the same with my word. I send it out, and it always produces fruit. It will accomplish all I want it to, and it will prosper everywhere I send it.* 1 Peter 1:23 says, *Being born again, not of corruptible seed, but of incorruptible, by the Word of God, which liveth and abideth for ever.* Luke 1:37 (AMP): *For with God nothing is ever impossible and no word from God shall be without power or impossible of fulfillment.*

May the Lord grant you a good and fertile heart to receive the living seed of His Word, and may the manifestation of your healing (the fruit of this Word) spring forth speedily.

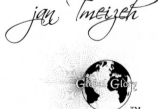

*Psalms 118:17 I shall not die, but live,
and declare the works of the Lord.*

Firm Foundation

A way for all

The Lord has graciously provided several ways for His people to receive healing. Of course, the way we all prefer it is when the healing power flows through our bodies and we receive a miraculous and immediate manifestation of healing. However, maybe you cannot get to a meeting where an anointed person can pray for you or lay hands on you; or maybe you are not associated with a church that has a pastor or believing elders who can anoint you with oil and pray the prayer of faith. Perhaps you are a new Believer, or one who has not received the proper teaching on healing. There could be any number of other reasons why at this point you may not be enjoying abundant health and life. I want to introduce you to a way that is available to all, all the time. It is not the easiest way, but it is one that is absolutely, positively guaranteed a healing outcome, regardless of the illness. Even people who have been declared hopeless have used this method and lived. People in desperate situations, even those who have been in accidents, have miraculously recovered. Simply stated, what I am referring to, is acquiring faith to be healed through hearing, meditating on, and speaking the Word of God.

This way requires some diligence and persistence. It has the side effects of developing character; producing some fruits of the Spirit, such as faith, patience, and self control; growth in the Spirit that cannot come any other way. It will develop love and compassion for others. It may even grow your faith to a level that will bring more immediate results for yourself and others in the future. You can develop such a strong, firm foundation in your belief in the Lord's provision for healing that you can never again be shaken.

PLEASE DO NOT PROCEED WITHOUT READING AND APPLYING THESE INSTRUCTIONS

There are some prerequisites, some preparatory steps, that must be taken at the outset to assure success. These are foundational, and without these properly in place, you proceed at your own risk. Why waste precious time?

WHO ARE YOU?

The first step is to know that you know, have the assurance in your heart, that you are a Christian. Until you know this as fact, it is futile to proceed, as everything you try to do will at most be temporary patch-work. It will merely affect the outward, the surface, the superficial; only to be lost in the end.

To be a Christian or Believer, you must be "born again." What does that mean? Is it simply believing that Jesus is the Son of God? Scripture tells us the demons believe and they tremble, and they are certainly not born again. If your mom and dad are or were Christians, does that make you one? If you are baptized into the church, does that mean you are a Christian? If you go to church and say the Lord's Prayer, and live a "good" life, does that make you a Christian? The answer is "no" to all of the above questions. Not even calling yourself a Christian makes you a Christian. Jesus said you, *individual you*, must be born again. That means born of the Spirit. He said, "I will give you a new heart," meaning a <u>new</u> <u>spirit</u>. He said, "I will dwell in you." Is He living, dwelling, abiding, having His home, His residence in you, inside your body, or are you alone living in your body? Who? Do you just let Him come and visit on Sunday mornings and that's it? Becoming a true Believer requires more than that. To experience this "new birth," the Bible gives us instructions as to what to do.

If you are a person who is seeking to know the truth about God, whose heart is longing for true freedom, whose soul is hurting, or who is crying out for God's deliverance, He will not turn you away. He is waiting with arms outstretched. He will receive you if you will but humble yourself, repent of your sins, repent of doing things your own way, with your own thoughts, your own will; give up your own ways and be willing to do everything His way, whatever it takes. He is waiting to fill you with His Spirit, with His power to become a son of God. He wants to transform your heart to make you new. He wants to remove that mountain of sin, doubt, unbelief, depression, discouragement, despair. Let Jesus come in by the power of the Holy Spirit and take possession of you—you'll be a new creature, you won't even know yourself anymore. When you let Jesus come in, He makes your heart pure, forms in you a new nature, and gives you divine triumph over sin and self. You won't just be a person saved from sin, but saved from *your sins*—sanctified (cleansed, holy, and set apart) by His Blood. You see, Jesus *gave up* His own life, His own health, His own strength, all His own glorious ways; He miraculously *took on* all your sins and the sins of the whole world. He took your sicknesses, your diseases, your confusion. In exchange, He gave you His righteousness. 2 Corinthians 5:21, The Twofold New Testament, 1865, Rev. Thomas Sheldon Green: *Him Who knew not sin, on our behalf He* (God) *made* (Him) *a thing of sin, that we might become God's righteousness in Him.* He took all that you are in your sin so that you could become all that He is in His righteousness. This is an amazing miracle. Only God could decree and accomplish such a strange and unique act. Jesus was not born in sin; He had no sin. He had no evil in Him; He was perfect, absolutely pure and holy. Evil could not touch Him. Sin could not touch Him—*but it did*.

His selling out was your being bought back and brought back to union and oneness with God your Creator; holy, like in the Garden of Eden before man sinned. You can be reestablished as the offspring of *very* God. This is the *exchanged* life. The wages of sin is death. Sin brings death. In taking your sin into Himself He took death into Himself. He took the very sin nature of mankind on Himself so that anyone who receives what He did can have His nature, the very nature of God. His pure and unadulterated Blood was presented to God His Father, the Judge of all, as the supreme and final sacrifice, once and forevermore. If you will give Him your life, He will give you His life.

> "Being bought back" is what redemption really means.

THE CORNERSTONE

First of all, you need to *repent*. "Repent" means *change your mind*. If you truly believe the previous section, you are ready. It is a decision, a choosing; a commitment to follow God's instructions. In addition to believing the previous, you are deciding to believe that the Bible is God's Word to mankind and to you specifically. This repenting is a turning from your sins, from going your own way, and determining to go God's way. You are resolving to turn your

"All Scripture is given by inspiration of God."

life over to His rulership, His authority. Ask Him to please forgive you for all your sins, to cleanse you of all unrighteousness, to please receive you into His kingdom, and fill you with His Spirit. Ask Him to please come inside you to live, to take up residence; to rule in your body; to rule over your mind, your thoughts, your emotions, your will.

God is a spirit. You cannot know Him through your mind; He can only be intimately known through your spirit. To have this knowledge, you must become like a child, and believe that Jesus is the *Sent One* from the heavenly realm, to show you how to know God your Father. Believe that He died, and was resurrected to give you life in the Spirit, and life forever. When He comes into your spirit, you can then understand spiritual things, and know His love, and the love of your Father.

A PRAYER FOR A NEW LIFE:
You may receive healing and deliverance immediately upon praying this prayer.

Father in Heaven, I believe You are the Creator of the universe and You are holy. I believe You sent Your only Son Jesus into the world. I believe He is the only true Messiah, the "Sent One." I believe the Bible is Your Word to mankind, and to me. I come to You admitting that I am a sinner; I have gone my own way; I have sinned. I am sorry for all that I have done wrong. I ask You to please forgive me. I am choosing to turn away from all sin and from every form of ungodliness. I believe that Your Son Jesus died on the cross as a final sacrifice and that His holy Blood cleanses me from all sin. I believe that You raised Him from the dead. I call upon Jesus the Messiah to be Lord and King over me. Jesus, I choose to die to myself and follow You all the days of my life. I ask that You fill me with the power of Your Holy Spirit. I declare that now I am a child of God and my life is not my own any longer. You have freed me from sin and made me the righteousness of God. I thank You that I have passed from hell into Heaven; from the kingdom of darkness into the Kingdom of Light; that You have lifted me out of death into life. I pray this in Jesus' name. Amen.

The next step is to confess Him with your mouth. Confession to another person is important in order to confirm your salvation. It says in Romans 10:9,10: *That if thou shalt confess with thy mouth the Lord Jesus, and shalt believe in thine heart that God hath raised Him from the dead, thou shalt be saved. For with the heart man believeth unto righteousness; and with the mouth confession is made unto salvation.*

Begin practicing obedience in all He wants you to do. You find out more by reading His Instruction Manual—the Bible. With His Spirit now inside, it will come alive to you and you will begin to understand it. See for yourself what He says. Talk to Him in prayer and throughout the day. Jesus will come in, fill your heart with peace and joy like you've never known, and give you a whole new life and purpose. Ask Him to direct you to a church in your area where you can be baptized in water (in obedience to His command), learn and grow, and be baptized in the Holy Spirit to receive power to live a holy life and to be His witness.

Jesus said, "I sanctify Myself." He *willfully* set Himself apart—deliberately.

DAILY PRAYER OF CONSECRATION:

Lord, I turn myself over to You. Fill me with Your Spirit. Guide me by Your Spirit. Give me a hunger for Your Word and help me to understand it. Manifest Your Spirit in me, to me, and through me, so that I may live a pure and obedient life today; that I may be Your witness today; that I may grow in You and operate in Your love today. Grant that I may live for Your glory. In Jesus' name, amen.

Proverbs 3:6 *Acknowledge the Lord in ALL your ways, and He will direct your paths.*

Translated

*Colossians 1:13 Who delivered us out of
the power of darkness, and translated
us into the kingdom
of His dear Son.*

WHO ARE YOU NOW?

After His Holy Spirit comes inside you, you are now *born anew*. With His Spirit, you are able to submit to Him as your King. That means you acknowledge Jesus and Jesus alone as King, *your* King. You must realize you are giving up your own worldly citizenship and becoming a citizen of Heaven where He rules supreme; He and not you any longer. This is for right now, here on this earth. The Kingdom of Heaven is inside you, Jesus said. You are now His ambassador on the earth. You take your orders from Him from now on.

Furthermore, though you still live in the world, you are no longer subject to many of the principles of the world. The curse is part of the world. It came into the world when Adam and Eve sinned. The Bible teaches that sickness and disease are part of the curse, and Jesus *became* that curse for us. The grip of the curse is broken when we are transferred into a different kingdom—the Kingdom of God. You are now delivered out from under the curse. There is no sickness and no disease in the Kingdom of God. Jesus was beaten with 39 stripes to break the curse of sickness. In 1 Peter 2:24, it says Jesus bore our sins in His body on the tree, and by His stripes we were healed. In Isaiah 53:4, the original Hebrew absolutely means *physical sickness* and *disease*. The Hebrew word *khali*, translated "griefs" in some versions, is never used for "sin"; it means *sickness* and *physical pain.* Matthew 8:17 confirms Jesus took our physical ailments upon Himself because it says that in fulfillment of Isaiah the prophet, He "took our *infirmities*, and bare our *sicknesses.*" Therefore, how could anyone believe that sickness or disease could possibly be God's will? Believing sickness is God's will is like saying Jesus took those stripes for nothing, or denying that He took the stripes, or denying that He fulfilled the prophecy.

The very word *salvation* includes healing. *Salvation* in the original Greek is *sotayria*—rescue or safety (physically or morally), and is translated "deliver," "health," "salvation," "save," "saving." When you have the new birth experience, you are in the domain of salvation. When you accepted Jesus, you accepted *all* that He did for you, the whole redemption package.

Y ou now have a new nature—a divine nature. (2 Corinthians 5:17, 2 Peter 1:4)

1 John 4:17b *As He is, so are we in this world.*

We are to be *like* God—to be conformed to the image of Jesus. Jesus said, "when you've seen Me, you've seen the Father." So we in turn are commanded to show the world Jesus. We are to prove to the world the power of prayer, the power of God's Word, the power of our God. This is what it means to be His witnesses. He commanded us to go forth, preach the Gospel, heal the sick, raise the dead, and cast out demons. Thus, after you are saved, you need the additional experience of being baptized (fully immersed) in the Holy Spirit; the *enduing with power*. All Believers are supposed to be revealing to the world that Jesus is the only way to knowing *intimately* God the Father, the Creator of the universe. We are to show forth the glory of the Lord! We have a relationship with the Almighty Creator and with His Son, through His Spirit. Christianity is not a religion like other religions. God is real. We _know_—we don't just think it—we know Him, we can hear Him, and we can feel Him. Anyone with a sincere heart, searching for the truth, will find it. If you seek Him with your whole heart, and stop looking to yourself and looking to things on the earth to fulfill you, He will manifest Himself to you. Look up! Look up unto Jesus! Look up to the Glorified One. Look into the heavenly realm where He is, the risen, reigning, glorified Son of God. He has been exalted to sit at the right hand of the throne of God; with all power, with the keys of hell and death—the divine authority, the eternal over-coming, the ultimate manifestation of God. Look up and let Him possess what He paid for—you!

YOU HAVE MOVED

Having given yourself wholly to Jesus now, you are in a new kingdom with new laws. There are spiritual principles and laws that are set and established by the Lord for Believers (Christians). Like the law of gravity is a physical principle or law, these are spiritual principles, and unchangeable. We must learn about these new laws and the ways of our King, in order to really know Him. To honor your new King, you must learn what pleases Him. The Bible says, "without faith it is impossible to please Him." That means faith is paramount to pleasing God. It is essential, and it tops the list of actions or ways that please Him. In actuality, without faith none of the other good deeds—not even love—will mean anything to God, because it would be nothing more than a human love without faith. You cannot *truly* love the Lord or your neighbor without faith; so you cannot fulfill the greatest commandment without faith. The reason being, before you can love God with all your heart, soul, strength, and mind, you must *believe* or *have the faith* that He *is*, that He exists. Actually, everything in this kingdom operates by the law of faith. So we as Believers must learn to function *by faith*. Four times in the Holy Scriptures the Lord says, *The just shall live by faith*. We learn to do this by renewing our minds, which will be discussed in the next section.

As a newborn person, you are equipped with all you need to succeed. However, you are just like a baby. You have all the right equipment, but you have to learn and grow; to come to know what it is that you have, and how to use what you have. The Bible says, to each is given a measure of faith. In order to mature as a child of God, your faith must grow. Like a child's legs must be used and exercised to get strong, so must your faith be used and exercised to become strong. Use it! You have nothing to lose but your doubt, and all to gain.

Faith

What is faith? How do we get it?
What do we do with it?

WHAT IS FAITH?

This kingdom is an unseen kingdom. God is not seen; Jesus is not seen; the Holy Spirit is not seen. Faith, abundant life, health, love, hope, peace, joy, ... all these are unseen, but they are indeed a part of this kingdom. James 1:17 says: *Every good gift and every perfect gift is from above, and comes down from the Father of Lights.* He desires for us to partake of all these blessings. Faith is the substance, the stuff, of these unseen gifts. Hebrews 11:1 (KJV)

> Faith is reaching out to what isn't there, and holding on till it is.

tells us: *Now faith is the substance of things hoped for, the evidence of things not seen.* Most of the translations use the word "assurance" here instead of "substance," but the original Greek word means: "a setting under (support)"; "concrete essence." Faith is the raw material, the stuff, of the things you desire that you do not yet see. Faith is believing what you do not see in the natural. Jesus told His disciples to pray: Thy kingdom come on earth—the same as it is in Heaven. So God wants all that He has provided to take on substance, to be made manifest, to come into being here on earth. Verse 3 of this same chapter tells us the world was put together by the Word of God, and that all that is seen was made out of unseen substance. It is through faith that we receive all the marvelous gifts and assets of our new kingdom.

> "Give us this day our daily bread" - Healing is the children's bread. (Mark 7:27)

> Things which we see were not made of things which we see.

HOW DO WE GET FAITH?

First of all, we cannot attain faith without renewing our minds. As a matter of fact, we have now come to the next level of our foundation: *the renewing of the mind*. When you are "born again" or "saved," it means you are born of the Spirit. Your spirit is all brand new, a whole new creation. 2 Corinthians 5:17 reads: *Therefore if any man be in Christ, he is a new creature: old things are passed away; behold, all things are become new.* Now if you died right away, you would immediately go to Heaven, and all would be well. There you would learn how everything operates according to a different set of laws.

Ephesians 4:23 "And be renewed in the spirit of your mind."

However, now you are still here on this earth, stuck with the same ol' mind and the same ol' body. This kingdom is inside you, in your spirit, and Jesus wants His kingdom, with all its benefits, brought into this earth, *right here, right now, through you.* For this to be possible we must undertake the renewing of the mind.

HOW DO WE DO THAT AND WHY IS IT SO IMPORTANT?

Renewing the mind is vital to gaining faith in order to receive all the benefits of God's kingdom, and for living a life fully for the Lord. It is the process by which we are conformed to His image. As we learn to think with a new mind, *the mind of Christ,* we will learn to create a world around ourselves full of kingdom manifestations. Faith, healing, and divine health are all part of living in the resurrected life of our King.

Romans 12:2 *And be not conformed to this world: but be ye transformed by the renewing of your mind, that ye may prove what is that good, and acceptable, and perfect, will of God.*

Colossians 3:10 *And have put on the new man, which is renewed in knowledge after the image of Him that created him.*

Philippians 2:5 *Let this mind be in you, which was also in Christ Jesus.*

You cannot grow in faith without renewing your mind. You cannot walk in divine healing without it. You cannot have true prosperity or wisdom without it. You cannot *know* "Truth" without it. Jesus said if you continue in His Word, you will be free—from sin,

Jesus said in John 8:31,32 "If you continue in My Word, you shall know the Truth and the Truth shall make you Free."

sickness, addictions; anything that does not belong in the kingdom. Continuing in His Word requires effort on a daily basis.

As we are continuing, our minds are being renewed, and faith is growing. Romans 10:17 says that *faith comes by hearing, and hearing by the Word of God.* It is the Word of God, the Bible, that is the key to renewing our minds and gaining faith so we can be victorious, healed, successful, fulfilled, and filled full of the power of God. When we walk in wholeness, with a new mind and a restored body, we reveal to the world that God's Word is Truth. But what does "continuing" really mean? I know people that read the Bible every day of their lives and do not live in

In the Greek, "Faith comes by hearing," indicates to hear and hear and hear, or a continual hearing.

victory or they are still sick. I know scholars that have studied it and also memorized it in Hebrew that are not even born again, much less know how to get healed. You cannot simply read it like a history book or a magazine. You must hear it with your spiritual ears; hear and hear and hear.

Prepare your mind for healing

Seeds must be rooted by watering before they can bring forth a harvest. The enemy wants to steal the Word before it is firmly rooted. Words do not get rooted, grow in the heart and bear fruit by just reading

Faith is expecting God to keep His promises.

them, but by meditating on them; giving deliberate thought and wholehearted attention to them. God has designed it so that when we hear and *meditate* on His Words about whatever promise that we need, faith arises in our hearts to receive that promise for ourselves. Herein is another of the spiritual laws of the Kingdom of God.

> Psalms 1:2,3 *His delight is in the Word of the Lord; and in His Word he <u>meditates</u> day and night. And he shall be like a tree <u>planted</u> by the rivers of water, that <u>brings forth</u> his <u>fruit</u> in his season; his leaf also shall not wither; and whatsoever he does shall prosper.*

> Joshua 1:8 *This book of the law shall not depart out of thy mouth; but thou shalt <u>meditate</u> therein day and night, that thou*

mayest observe to do according to all that is written therein: for <u>then</u> thou shalt make thy way prosperous, and <u>then</u> thou shalt have good success.

Meditation means *to dwell upon.* If you hear something over and over and over and think about it long enough, it will get down into your heart, your spirit. As a man thinketh in his heart, so is he. The word "meditation" connotes "rumination," which means "to ponder and turn over and over in the mind." In other words, to put forth effort to continually focus on a matter. *Noah Webster's New International Dictionary of the English Language* gives another very enlightening meaning to the word meditate. It says, "to purpose; to intend; to design; to plan by revolving in the mind." Meditate does not simply mean thinking about something, but planning and designing it in your **Meditate - Plan with a Purpose** mind with the intent that it will come to pass in your life. This is no doubt what God intended when He told us to do it.

WHAT DO WE DO WITH FAITH ONCE WE HAVE IT?

Faith is a tool to be used. Tools are used to do work; to fix things. The dictionary defines "tool" as *an implement for working*. It is the same with faith. Faith is a supernatural tool of the kingdom. It works in the heavenly realm as well as the earthly realm. Faith brings what you do not see into the physical world. It builds things, makes things, repairs things. In fact, through this incredible implement, anything and everything can be done. Through faith, nothing is impossible; i.e. <u>all</u> <u>things</u> <u>are</u> <u>possible</u>. Like a tool, it does nothing on its own, you must *work* it. Faith without working is dead. So how then do we *work* it?

Romans chapter 4 speaks about Abraham's faith being pleasing to God. His faith is what made him acceptable to God. It was his faith *working* that granted him the righteousness—not merely his faith in God, but his faith in *what God had spoken*. God had spoken the promise that Abraham would have a child. All evidence in the natural realm proved this to be an impossibility, but Abraham chose to believe God's Word.

Let there be no mistake about it. This chapter is not purely about Abraham gaining a right–standing with God. Note that Abraham was not believing in the promise in order to receive righteousness or to be accepted by God, even though that was one result of his believing. He was believing in the promise of a child, which was his desire. His faith was for the physical manifestation in the earth realm of a child being born in an impossible situation. It was the exercising, or *working* of his faith *by believing the Word of God* that caused God to be pleased with him *and* fulfill His promise.

KINGDOM WORK

Abraham put his faith in God's Word, without any physical evidence for it. Verse 17 says God *calls* those things which be not as though they were. God purposefully changed Abraham's name from *Abram* to *Abraham*, meaning "Father of Many Nations," so that every time his name was called, God's promise would be spoken forth. "Calling" means "speaking." More   **Calling = Speaking**
specifically, it means *to call forth by speaking out loud*. God speaks things that are impossible into

existence. Jesus said He does whatever He sees the Father doing. If we are to be conformed to His image, then we do likewise. Verses 23 and 24 say specifically that it was not written for Abraham's sake alone, but *for us* if we also believe.

So you see, speaking the Word, "calling" the Word, is one way of *working* your faith. Jesus told us to do it in Mark 11:23–24, when He said if you *say* and believe what you *say*, you shall have what you *say*. So He is teaching us that to operate your believing (your faith), you must *say* what you want. Another example is in Matthew 21:21, when He spoke to the fig tree and it yielded to the Word He had spoken. Throughout the Scriptures, we find many examples of this principle.

> God speaking, calling forth, is what brought the whole world into being. (Hebrews 11:3)

In the Gospel of St. Luke, chapter 17, verse 6, the Lord said, *If ye had faith as a grain of mustard seed, ye might say unto this sycamine tree, "Be thou plucked up by the root, and be thou planted in the sea"; and it should obey you.* That is an amazing statement; a great kingdom law, which allows us as Believers to speak to inanimate objects and have them do impossible things. Through faith they must obey what we say. Cancers, tumors, pains, fevers, all diseases have to obey our word.

Removing
Hindrances

The Bible has many promises, but they
are not without conditions.

Regardless of the malady, walking in divine health requires wisdom. Some sickness or disease is from sin; some from the devil; some simply because we live in a fallen world. The origin is not always clear. Therefore, I believe in covering all the bases.

First, ask the Lord if you need to repent for anything. He may bring something to mind. He may show you through the Word some disobedience, some situation where you have missed it. You may have neglected something He expects of you. If so, confess it, and ask His forgiveness and His help in making things right.

He may show you that you have some unforgiveness. You cannot expect to receive healing if
there is unforgiveness in your heart. Forgiving, no
matter how hard it may seem, is possible with His
help. You start by being willing, and praying in
earnest for Him to help you. If you are sincere, He
will reveal things to you; about yourself, or sometimes things about the other person that you did
not know. He may show you the state of their soul.
Then He may fill your heart with *His* love for them.
He may show you the state of your own heart, for
no matter what someone else has done to you, it
does not equal your sending the innocent man
Jesus to the cross. This may not be an easy process,
but it is absolutely mandatory; for He said plainly,
if we do not forgive, He will not forgive us.

Some sicknesses are a direct attack from the
devil and his evil cohorts. The Bible says the
devil goes about like a roaring lion, seeking whom
he may devour. It decrees Jesus went about doing
good and *healing all*
who were oppressed
by the devil. The

Hebrews 13:8 "Jesus Christ the same
yesterday, today, and Forever."

devil will take any opportunity to try to prove the

Blood of Jesus has no effect or has lost its power. Jesus was beaten for our healing, but the thief comes to steal all the good benefits provided us. The Word says satan comes to steal, to kill, and to destroy. The Lord Jesus gave us power over the devil. Luke 10:19 states, *Behold, I give unto you power to tread on serpents and scorpions, and over all the power of the enemy: and nothing shall by any means hurt you.* Jesus is our example. When He was tempted, after quoting the written Word, He spoke directly to satan and commanded him to leave. And in many instances He rebuked the *works* of the devil. Peter's mother–in–law is one example of this when Jesus "rebuked" the fever. 1 John 3:8 says Jesus was manifested for this purpose—to destroy the works of the devil. He is still the same and wants to accomplish that through us.

We need to take authority over the devil and his works by directly addressing him as Jesus did, *out loud*, commanding him in the name of Jesus to take his evil work off of our bodies. You cannot rebuke him in your mind; a command must be spoken. The Lord impressed upon me to give you more explicit instructions with a simple example.

If the flu is your mountain (see Mark 11:23), say:

> *In the name of the Lord Jesus, and by the authority of the Blood of Jesus, I command this flu to leave my body; satan, you take your flu and get out! You have no right to put sickness or disease on me. For it is written, "By His stripes I am healed." You are trespassing in my body. It is written, "I am a member of His body, of His flesh, and of His bones." Therefore no sickness or disease can be in my body because there is no sickness or disease, or any kind of infirmity in Jesus' body. Thank You Jesus that I am healed! ...*

The Word is our sword (Ephesians 6:17) and there are times it must be used as such. You cannot hide from the devil and expect any victory. You must take the offensive and use the sword of the Word by

Reading the Word out loud also dispels demons.

proclaiming it out of your mouth. If you are a meek and quiet person this may take quite a bit of effort.

Even if you are not, at times you may feel as if the devil has a muzzle over your mouth. You must overcome this. Continue battling with the Word multiple times per day until you see results. Some people will not receive their healing simply because they refuse to do this one thing. I heard someone say the devil is like an old stray dog following you down the road. You turn and say calmly, "Go on home now." The dog will pause, but as soon as you turn around he will continue following. You stop and turn again to say in a sterner voice, "Go home." He looks up at you pathetically, but as soon as you proceed, he continues right along. Finally, you turn, stomp your foot, and yell, *"Get out of here!"* at which point he hightails it away. The devil will test us to see if we seriously believe the Word of God, and will *enforce* the Word on him.

Just as it is very important to use your mouth to rebuke the devil, it is imperative to guard against speaking what is contrary to God's Word. This includes judging, criticizing, and complaining. It is especially dangerous to criticize ministers. Some of them may be in error or out of balance in certain areas, but most of them are trying to serve the Lord to the best of their knowledge and ability. It says in the Bible, "Speak evil of no man." It also says the devil is the accuser of the brethren. A fountain cannot bring forth fresh water and bitter (see James chapter 3). Proclaiming the Words of God to bring healing into your life cannot be mixed with speaking evil words.

> Psalms 39:1a *I said, I will take heed to my ways, that I sin not with my tongue: I will keep my mouth with a bridle.*

While you are busy declaring the healing Scriptures with your mouth, be sure you are not claiming the illness at the same time by saying, "*my* arthritis, *my* cancer, etc." If you are confessing the Word of healing and the symptoms at the same time, you are being double–minded.

Sometimes you must *contend* for your healing. I have seen people be touched by the Lord in a mighty way in a meeting and receive their healing. In the next day or so, or later that night, sometimes even before they leave the building, their symptoms return and they begin to doubt. This is the beginning of a battle. If the devil can get your mind focused on what you are feeling, then a door is opened for the sickness to return. At this point, you must take up your shield of faith to quench these fiery darts. You *must* take a stand and resist. Stand your ground by saying, "NO! devil I will not put up with your lying symptoms! I am healed and I am going to stay healed! So be gone from me in Jesus' name!" You may have to continue this kind of talk until the symptoms disappear, quoting the Word along with it.

Jonah 2:8 "They that observe lying vanities forsake their own mercy."

Likewise, your actions should show the devil you mean business. Act like a healed person!

Another stumbling block that will cause sickness and disease, and hinder healing is disobeying the natural laws that God laid out in the beginning. When He created our bodies, He made them to require food and rest. Our bodies must have certain amounts of nutrients in the proper combination to function. In the West, <u>most disease is a direct result of eating bad food</u>. In the beginning God made our bodies to live forever on fresh fruits and other plants. Only after sin came in did man begin to kill and eat meat. Now I am not saying we should all be vegetarians, although the Bible indicates some should; some people function better that way. Sometimes a serious illness calls for drastic measures. A life–threatening disease, for instance, should be treated differently than a cold. How can you expect to be restored to health if you continue to do the same things that caused the disease or problem in the first place? I have known and heard of many people with cancer and many other diseases who ate only fresh raw fruits and veggies, juiced, and were cured. If you have a major disease, the Lord expects you to make major changes in your lifestyle. A

> Proverbs 23:1-3 (NASB) "When you sit down to dine with a ruler, consider carefully what is before you, and put a knife to your throat if you are a man of great appetite – (NIV) if you are given to gluttony. Do not crave his delicacies, for that food is deceptive."

healthy lifestyle is also an important key to *keeping* your healing. If the Lord miraculously heals you and you go back to the same bad habits, you are very likely to lose your healing. The Word says your body is God's temple. You would not dump a bunch of trash in a church house; why pollute the real temple with junk food? I have studied nutrition for over 40 years, and have found that the best diet for *normal maintenance* is a well–balanced one. However, if you are sick or diseased, merely a well–balanced diet is not going to fix the problem.

Some people are in bondage to certain types of foods. This can be caused by fungus, diabetes, certain cancers and tumors, and other disorders. These cause people to crave substances that feed the disease. This, and bondage to other bad substances may require a regimen of fasting and herbs to cleanse your body and eliminate the disease–causing organisms. Studies have shown, and Scripture agrees, that fasting itself often brings restoration to health. Besides that, Jesus commands us to fast. He said "*when* you fast," not "*if* you fast."

A dequate sleep is necessary for good health. Even Jesus had to sleep. He got tired. He must have been extremely tired to sleep in a boat during a storm. I know; I used to work on a large sailboat and it was nearly impossible to sleep during a storm; and the smaller the boat, the worse it is. You must not deprive yourself, for the Bible says, "He gives His beloved sleep." Fresh air, plenty of good water, and exercise also have their place in healthy living.

The Bible teaches temperance and discipline in all areas of our lives. The Lord is more than willing to help us if we are failing in this area. But we must be willing to do our part, as well. Exercise your own will to try and keep trying. Above all else, <u>NEVER</u> <u>NEVER</u> <u>NEVER</u> give up! You may need to repent and pray for deliverance from bad eating habits, and of not taking the proper care for your body.

Furthermore, keep an attitude of expectancy. You could receive the manifestation of your healing at any time in any way. I suggest you pray with every minister who is offering prayer for healing, whether it be through TV, internet, other media, or in person. Even one word or phrase can be enough. God has innumerable ways of speaking to you. Years ago, when I was struggling with many physical problems, I had a turnaround in my own life and

Live in expectation!

health after my friend spoke a word straight from the Spirit into me: "Let's *live*, Jani—at least until we find out if He wants us to or not!" I found out! He *always* wants us to live! This unusual word from the Lord went directly into my soul, dispelled the doubt, and brought deliverance and release. Keep an open mind. Take the limits off of God. The Lord heals people in thousands of different ways. Remember He even used a donkey to speak His Word to someone! (Numbers 22)

Praise and worship create an atmosphere of expectancy. Praise puts power behind your faith. Some people receive their healing simply by praising and worshiping the Lord. Still others receive their healing by promising the Lord they will be His witness. But however you receive your healing, being thankful and testifying about it are still requirements. The Word of God says we are to live to the praise of His glory. It gives God **Have a thankful heart!** glory when we walk in health and share with people about His healing power. Moreover, it helps others in their fight of faith. We overcome by the Blood of the Lamb and the *word* of our testimony. The first part was His; the second part is ours. He has paid all for your all; He is worthy of highest glory, honor, and praise. Promise the Lord you will give Him all the glory and witness to others about your healing.

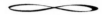

Counterattack

Don't be moved!

T his chapter I wrote as an addition when I thought the book was already finished. I felt the Lord was urging me by His Spirit to issue a warning so that when you are in the midst of a battle and feel as if you are losing, you will realize what is happening and you will not give up.

I am writing this from experience to provide you with more detail about the process you might go through when you decide you are going to contend for your healing. When you are attacked, you must launch an all–out counterattack. Intense pain wreaks havoc on your mental and emotional state. So does any serious disease. You may be confronted with fear, anger, frustration, self–pity, helplessness, hopelessness, depression, despair, and a gamut of other negative emotions. The devil starts his lies, which you must resist: "It won't work for you. It won't work this time. It's never been this bad. You're going to die. It's your time to die. Everyone would be better off without you ..." These thoughts are *not* from the Lord. They come directly to your mind from the devil, your own habitual way of thinking, or by negative words spoken through people. Refuse to entertain them. Also, do not allow yourself to get into reasoning—"Why did this happen? Why did You allow it to happen? If I hadn't done that, this wouldn't have happened. Are You punishing me? Don't You care? Are You even hearing me? ..." Focusing on these detrimental thoughts delays the process, gets your mind off the truth of God's Word, and brings confusion. The Word will dispel all of these. The quicker you get on the Scriptures and launch your counterattack, the quicker that Word will manifest in your flesh.

Pain is our enemy. It is part of the curse. It can, however, cause a person to become desperate enough to believe the Word and to do whatever it takes to be healed. During pain, you often think of the Lord and His suffering. It should make you feel compassion for others you may know who have suffered greatly. You become willing to repent of anything you may have done to offend the Lord or anyone else. Pain is a horrible ruthless enemy, cruel and pitiless. The Lord and His Word are the only forces that can cause any good to come from it.

I stated at the beginning this way is not the easiest, but there are occasions when there is no alternative. To use this method, you have to *really* want to be healed. Sometimes it can be very hard, depending on the seriousness of the situation, the amount of pain, the greatness of the attack. I have at times had to literally grit my teeth and speak the Word through tears and groans for days. If all the benefits of the kingdom always came easily, there would be no "pressing in" and we would not achieve full potential. It is the trials of our faith and the victories we obtain through *using the Word* during those trials that make us powerful and unshakable.

It is through *use* of, or as I specified before, *working*, the Word of God whereby you become mighty in faith, and maintain victory and stability in your life. For this is the victory that overcomes the world, even our faith. (1 Jn 5:4b) The word *overcome* itself entails an obstacle or a battle—you cannot overcome without a battle. *The world* here means all the natural forces that work against us, like diseases, pain, decay, our own minds, and the prince of this world, namely, the devil. Our enemy hates the Word of the Lord, and will try to keep you

"Take the Sword of the Spirit, which is the Word of God." Ephesians 6:17

from it in any way he can. He knows when you get this Word *in you*, you will have power over him, and nothing will be impossible to you.

The Lord has healed me many times through standing on His promises. These Scriptures and others have delivered me out of scores of various situations. Submit yourself to the Lord and ask Him to infuse you with His supernatural strength for this endeavor. Praise Him for His Blood that has paid for your healing. Ask the Holy Spirit to help you be diligent and faithful. When you have a mouth–mess–up by speaking negatively, repent quickly and get right back on the Word. Remember life and death are in your tongue.

Jesus never fails! His Word never fails! He heals ALL my diseases! He heals ALL your diseases! His healing Words have come to life in my body many times. If you do not fight with the Sword of the Word, you are beating the air. If you fight with the Word, you will *always* triumph. The Lord's Word always works if you stick with it, having a sincere heart, seeking the Lord all the while, and promising to honor Him with all your life.

Don't give up!
Work the Word.
Press in.
Get the victory!

Resurrection Life

Get to Work!

Having all these basics taken care of, we have laid the proper foundation. Now you must hear and meditate on the following healing Scriptures by reading them out loud several times a day. Do this relentlessly until faith comes. Be assured that it will, because God promises it will, and He is forever faithful. Then you will continue to read them, *with faith*; "calling" them out so that they will come into manifestation. Power to bring them to pass is inherent in the Words. (Remember the seed—I hope you have read the preface to this book.) You do your work and the Holy Spirit will do His.

> The power of life and death are in the tongue – your tongue.
> (Proverbs 18:21)

It is time for you to be "pleasing" to God by letting Him see you *working* your faith tool; confident that the Holy Spirit will *give life* to God's Words spoken through your mouth. "Call" yourself well!

> Joshua 1:8 (NIV) *Keep this Book of the Law always on your lips; meditate on it day and night, so that you may be careful to do everything written in it. Then you will be prosperous and successful.*

Now it is time to *work* your faith. He *will* give life to His own Words! Receive the resurrection life that is in these Words!

Note: In addition to healing Scriptures, I have included others that prepare the heart, and also firm up the healing Scriptures, to help you attain an unshakable faith in God's Word for *all* your needs.

Ps 118:17 (KJV) I shall not die, but live, and declare the works of the Lord.

Is 55:11 (KJV) So shall My Word be that goeth forth out of My mouth: it shall not return unto Me void, but it shall accomplish that which I please, and it shall prosper in the thing whereto I sent it.

Ro 4:21b What God has promised, He is able to perform.

Nu 23:19 (AMP) God is not a man, that He should tell or act a lie, neither the son of man, that He should feel repentance or compunction [for what He has promised]. Has He said and shall He not do it? Or has He spoken and shall He not make it good?

He 6:18a (DRB) It is impossible for God to lie.

Ps 119:89 (NAB) Your word, Lord, stands forever; it is firm as the heavens.

He 4:12a The Word of God speaks— (AMP) is alive and full of power [making it active, operative, energizing, and effective].

Jn 6:63b (KJV) The Words that I speak unto you, they are spirit, and <u>they are life</u>.

Ps 119:49,50 (AMP) Remember [fervently] the word and promise to Your servant, in which You have caused me to hope. This is my comfort and consolation in my affliction: that Your word has revived me and given me life.

Ps 119:116 (KJV) Uphold me according unto Thy Word, that I may live: and let me not be ashamed of my hope.

Ps 138:2b You honor Your Word above Your Name.

Ps 107:20 (KJV) He sent His Word, and healed them, and delivered them from (ALL, out of ALL) their destructions.

Ps 107:20 (AMP) He sends forth His word and heals them and rescues them from the pit and destruction.

Ps 107:20 (NLT) He sent out his word and healed them, snatching them from the door of death.

Ps 102:20 (ESV) To hear the groans of the prisoners, to set free those who were doomed to die.

Ps 119:25b (KJV) Quicken Thou me according to Thy Word.** (make me alive)

Ps 119:25b (NLT) Revive me by your word.

Ps 119:25b (ESV) Give me life according to your word!

Ps 119:92,93 (NIV) If your law had not been my delight, I would have perished in my affliction. I will never forget your precepts, for by them you have preserved my life.

Ps 119:93b (AKJV) For <u>with</u> <u>them</u> You have quickened me.** (made me live)

Ps 119:92,93 If I did not take pleasure in Your Word, I would have died in my affliction. I will never forget Your Word, for by it You have renewed my life.

Ps 119:77 (KJV) Let Thy tender mercies come unto me, that I may live: for Thy law is my delight.

Ps 119:148,149 (KJV) Mine eyes prevent the night watches, that I might meditate in Thy Word. Hear my voice according unto Thy lovingkindness: O Lord, quicken me (make me alive) according to Thy judgment.

Ps 119:17 (KJV) Deal bountifully with Thy servant, that I may live, and keep Thy Word.

Le 18:5 (KJV) Ye shall therefore keep My statutes, and My judgments: which if a man do, he shall live in them: I am the Lord.

De 7:9 (KJV) Know therefore that the Lord thy God, He is God, the faithful God, which keepeth covenant and mercy with them that love Him and keep His commandments to a thousand generations.

Pr 4:20–23 (NEB) My son, attend to my speech; pay heed to my words; do not let them slip out of your mind; keep them close in your heart; for they are life to him who finds them; and health to his whole body. Guard your heart more than any treasure, for it is the source of all life.

Pr 4:23 (KJV) Keep thy heart with all diligence; for out of it are the issues of life.

Ps 69:32 (KJV) The humble shall see this, and be glad: and your heart shall live that seek God.
(No more heart trouble!)

Pr 17:22 (AKJV) A merry heart does good like a medicine: but a broken spirit dries the bones.

Pr 17:22 (AMP) A happy heart is good medicine and a cheerful mind works healing, but a broken spirit dries up the bones.

Pr 14:30 (AMP) A calm and undisturbed mind and heart are the life and health of the body, but envy, jealousy, and wrath are like rottenness of the bones.

Ps 119:11 (KJV) Thy Word have I hid in mine heart, that I might not sin against Thee.
(Laboring to get God's Word into your heart will keep you from sin.)

Pr 4:10–12 (NEB) Listen, my son, take my words to heart, and the years of your life shall be multiplied. I will guide you in the paths of wisdom and lead you in honest ways. As you walk you will not slip, and, if you run, nothing will bring you down.

Pr 3:1b,2 (KJV) Let thine heart keep My commandments: for length of days, and long life, and peace, shall they add to thee.

Pr 9:11 (KJV) For by me thy days shall be multiplied, and the years of thy life shall be increased.

Pr 9:11 (GW) You will live longer because of me, and years will be added to your life.

De 5:33 (NLT) Stay on the path that the LORD your God has commanded you to follow. Then you will live long and prosperous lives in the land you are about to enter and occupy.

Eph 6:1–3 (KJV) Children, obey your parents in the Lord: for this is right. Honor your father and mother; which is the first commandment with promise; that it may be well with you, and you may live long on the earth.

Je 29:11 I know the intentions I have for you, declares the Lord, plans for shalom—peace, good health, prosperity, wholeness, and not for calamity—affliction and distress; to give you a future full of expectancy.

De 30:19b (NASB) I have set before you life and death, the blessing and the curse. So choose life in order that you may live, you and your descendants.

De 30:19b (NASB) Choose life in order that you may live.

Re 22:17 (KJV) Whosoever will, let him take the water of life freely.

Jn 1:4a (KJV) In Him was life.

Ro 8:11 (KJV) But if the Spirit of Him that raised up Jesus from the dead dwell in you, He that raised up Christ from the dead shall also quicken (give life to) your mortal bodies by His Spirit that dwelleth in you.

Is 53:4,5 (KJV) Surely He hath borne our griefs, and carried our sorrows: yet we did esteem Him stricken, smitten of God, and afflicted. But He was wounded for our transgressions, He was bruised for our iniquities: the chastisement of our peace was upon Him; and with His stripes we are healed.

Is 53:4,5 (NEB) Yet on himself he bore our sufferings, our torments he endured, while we counted him smitten by God, struck down by disease and misery; but he was pierced for our transgressions, tortured for our iniquities; the chastisement he bore is health for us and by his scourging we are healed.

Is 53:4 He bore all our suffering and misery; He took on Himself our infirmities, our afflictions. He bore our sickness, weakness and pain. He was made sick with our sickfulness.

1Pt 2:24b (TCNT) His bruising was your healing.

Mt 8:17 (AMP) And thus He fulfilled what was spoken by the prophet Isaiah, He Himself took [in order to carry away] our weaknesses and infirmities and bore away our diseases.

Mt 8:17b Himself Jesus bore our infirmities and carried our diseases.

1Pt 2:24 (KJV) Who His own self bare our sins in His own body on the tree, that we, being dead to sins, should live unto righteousness: by Whose stripes ye were healed.

1Pt 2:24 (NASB) And He Himself bore our sins in His body on the cross, so that we might die to sin and live to righteousness; for by His wounds you were healed.

1Pt 2:24 (AMP) He personally bore our sins in His [own] body on the tree [as on an altar and offered Himself on it], that we might die (cease to exist) to sin and live to righteousness. By His wounds you have been healed.

1Pt 2:24b By His stripes we were healed.

1Pt 2:24b By His stripes I am healed.

Jb 33:24,25 (AMP) Then [God] is gracious to him and says, Deliver him from going down into the pit [of destruction]; I have found a ransom (a price of redemption, an atonement)! [Then the man's] flesh shall be restored; it becomes fresher and more tender than a child's; he returns to the days of his youth.

Je 33:6 (KJV) Behold, I will bring it health and cure, and I will cure them, and will reveal unto them the abundance of peace and truth.

Je 33:6 (NASB) Behold, I will bring to it health and healing, and I will heal them; and I will reveal to them an abundance of peace and truth.

Ex 15:26b (KJV) I am the Lord that healeth thee.

Ex 15:26b (ESV) For I am the LORD, your healer.

Mal 3:6a (KJV) For I am the Lord, I change not.

He 13:8 (KJV) Jesus Christ the same yesterday, and today, and forever.

Je 17:14 (KJV) Heal me, O Lord, and I shall be healed; save me, and I shall be saved: for Thou art my praise.

Ps 42:11b, 43:5b (KJV) Who is the health of my countenance, and my God.

Ps 105:37 (KJV) He brought them forth also with silver and gold: and there was not one feeble person among their tribes.

Ex 23:25 (KJV) And ye shall serve the Lord your God, and He shall bless thy bread, and thy water; and I will take sickness away from the midst of thee.

Is 58:8a (AMP) Then shall your light break forth like the morning, and your healing (your restoration and the power of a new life) shall spring forth speedily.
(Isaiah 58 is the fasting chapter.)

Ps 84:11b,12 (KJV) No good thing will He withhold from them that walk uprightly. O Lord of hosts, blessed is the man that trusteth in Thee.

Ps 37:4 (KJV) Delight thyself also in the Lord; and He shall give thee the desires of thine heart.

Jn 14:13,14 (KJV) And whatsoever ye shall ask in My Name, that will I do, that the Father may be glorified in the Son. If ye shall ask anything in My Name, I will do it.

Jn 16:23b,24b (KJV) Verily, verily, I say unto you, whatsoever ye shall ask the Father in My Name, He will give it you. Ask, and ye shall receive, that your joy may be full.

1Jn 3:22 (KJV) And whatsoever we ask, we receive of Him, because we keep His commandments, and do those things that are pleasing in His sight.

Mt 7:7, Lk 11:9 (KJV) Ask, and it shall be given you; seek, and ye shall find; knock, and it shall be opened unto you.

Jn 15:7 (GW) If you live in me and what I say lives in you, then ask for anything you want, and it will be yours.

Jn 15:7 (AMP) If you live in Me [abide vitally united to Me] and My words remain in you and continue to live in your hearts, ask whatever you will, and it shall be done for you.

Jn 14:12–14 (AMP) I assure you, most solemnly I tell you, if anyone steadfastly believes in Me, he will himself be able to do the things that I do; and he will do even greater things than these, because I go to the Father. And I will do [I Myself will grant] whatever you ask in My Name [as presenting all that I AM], so that the Father may be glorified and extolled in (through) the Son. [Yes] I will grant [I Myself will do for you] whatever you shall ask in My Name [as presenting all that I AM].

Eph 3:20 He is able to do exceeding abundantly above all that we ask or think, according to the power that works in us.

Eph 3:20,21 (AMP) Now to Him Who, by (in consequence of) the [action of His] power that is at work within us, is able to [carry out His purpose and] do superabundantly, far over and above all that we [dare] ask or think [infinitely beyond our highest prayers, desires, thoughts, hopes, or dreams]—To Him be glory in the church and in Christ Jesus throughout all generations forever and ever. Amen (so be it).

1Jn 5:14,15 (AKJV) And this is the confidence that we have in Him, that, if we ask any thing according to His will, He hears us: and if we know that He hear us, whatever we ask, we know that we have the petitions that we desired of Him.

Mk 11:24 That is why I tell you, whatever you desire, whatever you pray about and ask for, believe that you receive them; you will receive, you have received, and you shall have them.

Mk 11:24–26 Therefore I say unto you, whatever things you desire, when you pray, believe that you receive them, (AMP) (trust and be confident) that it is granted to you, and you will [get it]. And whenever you stand praying, if you have anything against anyone, forgive him and let it drop (leave it, let it go), in order that your Father Who is in heaven may also forgive you your [own] failings and shortcomings and let them drop. But if you do not forgive, neither will your Father in heaven forgive your failings and shortcomings.

Eph 4:32 (KJV) And be ye kind one to another, tenderhearted, forgiving one another, even as God for Christ's sake hath forgiven you.

1Jn 1:9 (AMP) If we [freely] admit that we have sinned and confess our sins, He is faithful and just (true to His own nature and promises) and will forgive our sins [dismiss our lawlessness] and [continuously] cleanse us from all unrighteousness [everything not in conformity to His will in purpose, thought, and action].

1Jn 1:9 (KJV) If we confess our sins, He is faithful and just to forgive us our sins, and to cleanse us from all unrighteousness.

Ps 32:5b After confession, You removed my guilt.

Ps 86:5 (KJV) For Thou, Lord, art good, and ready to forgive; and plenteous in mercy unto all them that call upon Thee.

Ps 103:3 (KJV) Who forgiveth all thine iniquities; Who healeth all thy diseases. (ALL!)

Ps 103:1–3 (NEB) Bless the Lord, my soul; my innermost heart, bless his holy name. Bless the Lord, my soul, and forget none of his benefits. He pardons all my guilt and heals all my suffering. (ALL!)

Ro 8:1,2 (AMP) Therefore, [there is] now no condemnation (no adjudging guilty of wrong) for those who are in Christ Jesus, who live [and] walk not after the dictates of the flesh, but after the dictates of the Spirit. For the law of the Spirit of life [which is] in Christ Jesus [the law of our new being] has freed me from the law of sin and of death.

Ro 6:14a (KJV) Sin shall not have dominion over you.

Ga 3:13,14a (KJV) Christ hath redeemed us from the curse of the law, being made a curse for us: for it is written, Cursed is every one that hangeth on a tree: that the blessing of Abraham might come on the Gentiles through Jesus Christ.

Ga 3:29 If you are in Yeshua the Messiah, you are indeed Abraham's children, and you inherit all the promises.

Mk 7:27 Healing is the children's bread.

Ps 68:19a (KJV) Blessed be the Lord, who daily loadeth us with benefits. Is sickness a benefit? NO!

3Jn v2 (KJV) Beloved, I wish above all things that thou mayest prosper and be in health, even as thy soul prospereth.

3Jn v2 (AMP) Beloved, I pray that you may prosper in every way and [that your body] may keep well, even as [I know] your soul keeps well and prospers.

3Jn v2 (NIV) Dear friend, I pray that you may enjoy good health and that all may go well with you, even as your soul is getting along well.

Lk 6:19 (AMP) And all the multitude were seeking to touch Him, for healing power was all the while going forth from Him and curing them all [saving them from severe illnesses or calamities].

Mt 8:16 (KJV) When the even was come, they brought unto Him many that were possessed with devils: and He cast out the spirits with His Word, and healed ALL that were sick.

Lk 7:7b,9,10 (NLT) Just say the word from where you are, and my servant will be healed. When Jesus heard this, he was amazed. Turning to the crowd that was following him, he said, "I tell you, I haven't seen faith like this in all Israel!" And when the officer's friends returned to his house, they found the slave completely healed.

Mt 19:2 (KJV) Great multitudes followed Him; and He healed them there.

Mt 12:15b (KJV) Great multitudes followed Him, and He healed them ALL.
(Jesus healed everyone who asked. There were no exceptions.)

Mt 4:23 (AMP) And He went about all Galilee, teaching in their synagogues and preaching the good news (Gospel) of the kingdom, and healing every disease and every weakness and infirmity among the people.

Mt 11:5 (KJV) The blind receive their sight, and the lame walk, the lepers are cleansed, and the deaf hear, the dead are raised up, and the poor have the Gospel preached to them.

Mt 15:30 (KJV) And great multitudes came unto Him, having with them those that were lame, blind, dumb, maimed, and many others, and cast them down at Jesus' feet; and He healed them.

Mt 15:31 The people glorified the God of Israel when they saw the dumb speaking, the maimed be made whole, the lame walking, the blind seeing.

Mt 12:10a,13 (KJV) And, behold, there was a man which had his hand withered. Then saith He (Jesus) to the man, Stretch forth thine hand. And he stretched it forth; and it was restored whole, like as the other.

Mt 8:2,3a (KJV) And behold, there came a leper and worshipped Him, saying, Lord, if Thou wilt, Thou canst make me clean. And Jesus put forth His hand, and touched him, saying, I will; be thou clean.

"I will."

Mk 1:41 (KJV) And Jesus, moved with compassion, put forth His hand, and touched him, and saith unto him, I will; be thou clean.

"Absolutely I want to, be clean."

1Th 5:23 (KJV) The very God of peace sanctify you wholly; and I pray God your whole spirit and soul and body be preserved blameless unto the coming of our Lord Jesus Christ.

1Th 5:23 (AMP) And may the God of peace Himself sanctify you through and through [separate you from profane things, make you pure and wholly consecrated to God]; and may your spirit and soul and body be preserved sound and complete [and found] blameless at the coming of our Lord Jesus Christ (the Messiah).

Ps 30:2 (AKJV) O Lord my God, I cried to You, and You have healed me.

Mal 4:2a (KJV) But unto you that fear My Name shall the Sun of Righteousness arise with healing in His wings.

De 7:15a (KJV) And the Lord will take away from thee all sickness, and will put none of the evil diseases of Egypt, which thou knowest, upon thee. (He said He wouldn't under the Old Covenant; how much less under the New.)

Je 30:17a (WEB) For I will restore health to you, and I will heal you of your wounds, says Yahweh.

Mt 9:27–30a (KJV) When Jesus departed thence, two blind men followed Him, crying, and saying, Thou Son of David, have mercy on us. And when He was come into the house, the blind men came to Him: and Jesus saith unto them, Believe ye that I am able to do this? They said unto Him, Yea, Lord. Then touched He their eyes, saying, According to your faith be it unto you. And their eyes were opened.

Lk 18:35b–43 (WNT, KJV) There was a blind man sitting by the way–side begging. He heard a crowd of people going past, and inquired what it all meant. "Jesus of Nazareth is passing by," they told him. Then, at the top of his voice, he cried out, "Jesus, son of David, have mercy on me." Those in front reproved him and tried to silence him; but he continued shouting, louder than ever, "Son of David, have mercy on me." At length Jesus stopped and desired them to bring the man to Him; and when he had come close to Him He asked him, "What shall I do for you?" "Sir," he replied, "that I may receive my sight." "Receive your sight," said Jesus: "your faith has cured you." No sooner were the words spoken than the man regained his sight and followed Jesus, giving glory to God; and all the people, seeing it, gave praise to God.

Lk 17:12–14 (AMP) And as He was going into one village, He was met by ten lepers, who stood at a distance. And they raised up their voices and called, Jesus, Master, take pity and have mercy on us! And when He saw them, He said to them, Go [at once] and show yourselves to the priests. And as they went, they were cured and made clean.

Jn 5:3a,5–9a (AMP) In these lay a great number of sick folk—some blind, some crippled, and some paralyzed (shriveled up)—There was a certain man there who had suffered with a deep–seated and lingering disorder for thirty–eight years. When Jesus noticed him lying there [helpless], knowing that he had already been a long time in that condition, He said to him, Do you want to become well? [Are you really in earnest about getting well?] The invalid answered, Sir, I have nobody when the water is moving to put me into the pool; but while I am trying to come [into it] myself, somebody else steps down ahead of me. Jesus said to him, Get up! Pick up your bed (sleeping pad) and walk! Instantly the man became well and recovered his strength and picked up his bed and walked.

Mt 20:30–34 (KJV) Behold, two blind men sitting by the wayside, when they heard that Jesus passed by, cried out, saying, Have mercy on us, O Lord, Thou Son of David, and the multitude rebuked them, because they should hold their peace: but they cried the more, saying, Have mercy on us, O Lord, Thou Son of David. And

Jesus stood still, and called them, and said, What will ye that I shall do unto you? They say unto Him, Lord, that our eyes may be opened. So Jesus had compassion on them, and touched their eyes: and immediately their eyes received sight, and they followed Him.

Jn 11:38–44 (NIV) Jesus, once more deeply moved, came to the tomb. It was a cave with a stone laid across the entrance. "Take away the stone," he said. "But, Lord," said Martha, the sister of the dead man, "by this time there is a bad odor, for he has been there four days." Then Jesus said, "Did I not tell you that if you believed, you will see the glory of God?" So they took away the stone. Then Jesus looked up and said, "Father, I thank you that you have heard me. I knew that you always hear me, but I said this for the benefit of the people standing here, that they may believe that you sent me." When he had said this, Jesus called in a loud voice, "Lazarus, come out!" The dead man came out, his hands and feet wrapped with strips of linen, and a cloth around his face. Jesus said to them, "Take off the grave clothes and let him go."

Mk 5:21–42a (NIV) When Jesus had again crossed over by boat to the other side of the lake, a large crowd gathered around him while he was by the lake. Then one of the synagogue leaders, named Jairus, came, and when he saw Jesus, he fell at his feet. He pleaded earnestly with him, "My little daughter is dying. Please come and put your hands on her so that she will be healed and live." So Jesus went with him. A large crowd followed and pressed around him. And a woman was there who had been subject to bleeding for twelve years. She had suffered a great deal under the care of many doctors and had spent all she had, yet instead of getting better she grew worse. When she heard about Jesus, she came up behind him in the crowd and touched his cloak, because she thought, "If I just touch his clothes, I will be healed." Immediately her bleeding stopped and she felt in her body that she was freed from her suffering. At once Jesus realized that power had gone out from him. He turned around in the crowd and asked, "Who touched my clothes?" "You see the people crowding against you," his disciples answered, "and yet you can ask, 'Who touched me?'" But Jesus kept looking around to see who had done it. Then the woman, knowing what had happened to her, came and fell at his feet and, trembling with fear, told him the whole truth. He said to her, "Daughter, your faith has healed you. Go in peace and be freed from your suffering." While Jesus was still speaking, some people came from the house of Jairus, the synagogue leader. "Your daughter is dead," they said. "Why bother the teacher anymore?" Overhearing what they said, Jesus told him, "Don't be afraid; just believe." He did not let anyone follow him except Peter, James and John the brother of James. When they came to the home of the synagogue leader, Jesus saw a commotion, with people crying and wailing loudly. He went in and said to them, "Why all this commotion and wailing? The child is not dead but asleep." But they laughed at him. After he put them all out, he took the child's father and mother and the disciples who were with him, and went in where the child was. He took her by the hand and said to her, "Talitha koum!" (which means "Little girl, I say to you, get up!"). Immediately the girl stood up and began to walk around (she was twelve years old).

Mt 9:35 (DBY) And Jesus went round all the cities and the villages, teaching in their synagogues, and preaching the glad tidings of the kingdom, and healing EVERY disease and EVERY bodily weakness.

He 13:8 (LEB) Jesus Christ is the same yesterday and today and forever.

Jm 1:17a (KJV) Every good gift and every perfect gift is from above, and cometh down from the Father.

Lk 11:13 (AMP) If you then, evil as you are, know how to give good gifts [gifts that are to their advantage] to your children, how much more will your heavenly Father give the Holy Spirit to those who ask and continue to ask Him!

Lk 4:18,19 (KJV) The Spirit of the Lord is upon Me, because He hath anointed Me to preach the Gospel to the poor; He hath sent Me to heal the brokenhearted, to preach deliverance to the captives, and recovering of sight to the blind, to set at liberty them that are bruised, to preach the acceptable year of the Lord.

Lk 4:18 The Spirit of the Lord is upon me, because He has anointed me to preach the Gospel to the afflicted; He has sent me to heal the brokenhearted, to preach deliverance to the captives, to announce to prisoners: you are free; recovering of sight to the blind, new eyes for the blind; to set at liberty them that are bruised (downtrodden); to free those who have been crushed by sin; (those who have been shattered through the ravages of sin).

Lk 9:2 He instructed them to preach the Kingdom of God and to heal the sick.

Mk 16:18b (KJV) They shall lay hands on the sick, and they shall recover.

Mk 16:17,18,20 (KJV) And these signs shall follow them that believe; In My Name shall they cast out devils; they shall speak with new tongues; they shall take up serpents; and if they drink any deadly thing, it shall not hurt them; they shall lay hands on the sick, and they shall recover. And they went forth, and preached everywhere, the Lord working with them, and confirming the Word with signs following. Amen. (so be it)

Mt 10:7,8 (KJV) And as ye go, preach, saying, The Kingdom of Heaven is at hand. Heal the sick, cleanse the lepers, raise the dead, cast out devils: freely ye have received, freely give.

Ac 5:16 (KJV) There came also a multitude out of the cities round about unto Jerusalem, bringing sick folks, and them which were vexed with unclean spirits: and they were healed EVERY ONE.

Mk 6:13 (KJV) And they cast out many devils, and anointed with oil many that were sick, and healed them.

Jm 5:14–16 (KJV) Is any sick among you? Let him call for the elders of the church; and let them pray over him, anointing him with oil in the Name of the Lord: and the prayer of faith shall save the sick, and the Lord shall raise him up; and if he have committed sins, they shall be forgiven him. (WNT) Therefore confess your sins to one another, and pray for one another, so that you may be cured. The heartfelt supplication of a righteous man exerts a mighty influence.

Ac 3:1–8 (KJV) Peter and John went up together into the temple at the hour of prayer, being the ninth hour. And a certain man lame from his mother's womb was carried, whom they laid daily at the gate of the temple which is called Beautiful, to ask alms of them that entered into the temple; who seeing Peter and John about to go into the temple asked an alms. And Peter, fastening his eyes upon him with John, said, Look on us. And he gave heed unto them, expecting to receive something of them. Then Peter said, Silver and gold have I none; but such as I have give I thee: in the Name of Jesus Christ of Nazareth rise up and walk. And he took him by the right hand, and lifted him up: and immediately his feet and ankle bones received strength. And he leaping up stood, and walked, and entered with them into the temple, walking, and leaping, and praising God.

Ac 9:32–34 (KJV) And it came to pass, as Peter passed throughout all quarters, he came down also to the saints which dwelt at Lydda. And there he found a certain man named Aeneas, which had kept his bed eight years, and was sick of the palsy. And Peter said unto him, Aeneas, Jesus Christ maketh thee whole: arise, and make thy bed. And he arose immediately.

Ac 14:8–10 (KJV) There sat a certain man at Lystra, impotent in his feet, being a cripple from his mother's womb, who never had walked: The same heard Paul speak: who steadfastly beholding him, and perceiving that he had faith to be healed, said with a loud voice, Stand upright on thy feet. And he leaped and walked.

Ac 8:5–7 (GW) Philip went to the city of Samaria and told people about the Messiah. The crowds paid close attention to what Philip said. They listened to him and saw the miracles that he performed. Evil spirits screamed as they came out of the many people they had possessed. Many paralyzed and lame people were cured.

Ac 19:11,12 (KJV) And God worked special miracles by the hands of Paul: so that from his body were brought unto the sick handkerchiefs or aprons, and the diseases departed from them, and the evil spirits went out of them.

(Yet another of the many ways you can be healed.)

Ps 121:7 (KJV) The Lord shall preserve thee from all evil: He shall preserve thy soul (life).

Ps 91:10,11 (KJV) There shall no evil befall thee, neither shall any plague come nigh thy dwelling. For He shall give His angels charge over thee, to keep thee in all thy ways.

Ps 91:1–4 (KJV) He that dwelleth in the secret place of the Most High shall abide under the shadow of the Almighty. I will say of the Lord, He is my refuge and my fortress: my God; in Him will I trust. Surely He shall deliver thee from the snare of the fowler, and from the noisome pestilence. He shall cover thee with His feathers, and under His wings shalt thou trust: His Truth shall be thy shield and buckler.

Pr 29:25b (KJV) Whoso putteth his trust in the Lord shall be safe.

Ps 118:6a (NIV) The LORD is with me; I will not be afraid.

Mk 5:36b (KJV) Be not afraid, only believe.

Is 26:3 (KJV) Thou wilt keep him in perfect peace, whose mind is stayed on Thee: because he trusteth in Thee.

Is 26:3 (NIV) You will keep in perfect peace those whose minds are steadfast, because they trust in you.

2Ti 1:7 (KJV) For God hath not given us the spirit of fear; but of power, and of love, and of a sound mind.

2Ti 1:7 (AMP) For God did not give us a spirit of timidity (of cowardice, of craven and cringing and fawning fear), but [He has given us a spirit] of power and of love and of calm and well–balanced mind and discipline and self–control.

Lk 12:7b Fear not, stop being afraid; you are more precious than many sparrows.

Is 41:10 (KJV) Fear thou not; for I am with thee: be not dismayed; for I am thy God: I will strengthen thee; yea, I will help thee; yea, I will uphold thee with the right hand of My righteousness.

Ps 46:1,2 (NASB) God is our refuge and strength, a very present help in trouble. Therefore we will not fear, though the earth should change and though the mountains slip into the heart of the sea.

Ps 27:1 (KJV) The Lord is my light and my salvation; whom shall I fear? The Lord is the strength of my life; of whom shall I be afraid?

Is 40:31 (KJV) But they that wait upon the Lord shall renew their strength; they shall mount up with wings as eagles; they shall run, and not be weary; and they shall walk, and not faint.

Ps 68:35 (AMP) O God, awe–inspiring, profoundly impressive, and terrible are You out of Your holy places; the God of Israel Himself gives strength and fullness of might to His people. Blessed be God!

Col 1:11a (KJV) Strengthened with all might, according to His glorious power.

Col 1:11 (NASB) Strengthened with all power, according to His glorious might, for the attaining of all steadfastness and patience; joyously.

Col 1:11a (WNT) Since His power is so glorious, may you be strengthened with strength of every kind.

Ps 29:11a (KJV) The Lord will give strength unto His people.

Ps 68:28a (NASB) Your God has commanded your strength.

Ps 41:1–3 (KJV) Blessed is he that considereth the poor: the Lord will deliver him in time of trouble. The Lord will preserve him, and keep him alive; and he shall be blessed upon the earth: and Thou wilt not deliver him unto the will of his enemies. The Lord will strengthen him upon the bed of languishing: Thou wilt make all his bed in his sickness.

Mi 3:8a (KJV) Truly I am full of power by the Spirit of the Lord, and of judgment, and of might (force, valor, victory, power, strength).

Is 40:29 (KJV) He giveth power to the faint; and to them that have no might He increaseth strength.

Is 40:29 (NEB) He gives vigor to the weary, new strength to the exhausted.

Ps 73:26b (KJV) God is the strength of my heart, and my portion for ever.

Joel 3:10b (KJV) Let the weak say, I am strong.
(Keep calling yourself well.)

Ro 14:4b The Lord is able to make me stand.

Ps 92:10 (GW) But you make me as strong as a wild bull, and soothing lotion is poured on me.

Ps 92:11 [92:10] (NAB)
You have given me the strength of a wild ox;
you have poured rich oil upon me.

Ps 71:16 (KJV) I will go in the strength of the Lord God: I will make mention of Thy righteousness, even of Thine only.

Is 26:4 Put your trust in the Mighty Almighty all your life; because He is a Rock of strength for you for now and always.

Pr 24:5 (KJV) A wise man is strong; yea, a man of knowledge increaseth strength.

Pr 3:7,8 (NLT) Don't be impressed with your own wisdom. Instead, fear the LORD and turn away from evil. Then you will have healing for your body and strength for your bones.

Ne 8:10b (KJV) For the joy of the Lord is your strength.

Eph 6:10 (NASB) Finally, be strong in the Lord and in the strength of His might.

Da 11:32b (KJV) The people that do know their God shall be strong, and do exploits.

Ph 4:13 (WEB) I can do all things through Christ, Who strengthens me.

Ps 8:2 (KJV) Out of the mouth of babes and sucklings hast Thou ordained strength because of Thine enemies, that Thou mightest still the enemy and the avenger.

Ac 10:38 (KJV) How God anointed Jesus of Nazareth with the Holy Ghost and with power: Who went about doing good, and healing ALL that were oppressed of the devil; for God was with Him.

Ac 10:38 (AMP) How God anointed and consecrated Jesus of Nazareth with the [Holy] Spirit and with strength and ability and power; how He went about doing good and, in particular, curing all who were harassed and oppressed by [the power of] the devil, for God was with Him.

Mt 12:22 (GW) Then some people brought Jesus a man possessed by a demon. The demon made the man blind and unable to talk. Jesus cured him so that he could talk and see.

Lk 13:11–13 (AMP) And there was a woman there who for eighteen years had had an infirmity caused by a spirit (a demon of sickness). She was bent completely forward and utterly unable to straighten herself up or to look upward. And when Jesus saw her, He called [her to Him] and said to her, Woman, you are released from your infirmity! Then He laid [His] hands on her, and instantly she was made straight, and she recognized and thanked and praised God.

Lk 13:16 (KJV) And ought not this woman, being a daughter of Abraham, whom satan hath bound, lo, these eighteen years, be loosed from this bond?

He 2:14 (NET) Therefore, since the children share in flesh and blood, he likewise shared in their humanity, so that through death he could destroy the one who holds the power of death (that is, the devil).

Jn 10:10 (AKJV) The thief comes not, but for to steal, and to kill, and to destroy: I am come that they might have life, and that they might have it more abundantly. (Overflowing)

Eph 6:10–12 (KJV) Be strong in the Lord, and in the power of His might. Put on the whole armour of God, that you may be able to stand against the wiles of the devil. For we wrestle not against flesh and blood, but against principalities, against powers, against the rulers of the darkness of this world, against spiritual wickedness in high places.

Eph 6:10–12 (AMP) In conclusion, be strong in the Lord [be empowered through your union with Him]; draw your strength from Him [that strength which His boundless might provides]. Put on God's whole armor [the armor of a heavy–armed soldier which God supplies], that you may be able successfully to stand up against [all] the strategies and the deceits of the devil. For we are not wrestling with flesh and blood [contending only with physical opponents], but against the despotisms, against the powers, against [the master spirits who are] the world rulers of this present darkness, against the spirit forces of wickedness in the heavenly (supernatural) sphere.

2Co 10:3–5 For although we live in the world it is no worldly warfare that we are waging. (AMP) For the weapons of our warfare are not physical [weapons of flesh and blood], but they are mighty before God for the overthrow and destruction of strongholds, (KJV) casting down imaginations, and every high thing that exalteth itself against the knowledge of God, and bringing into captivity every thought to the obedience of Christ.

Jm 4:7 (KJV) Submit yourselves therefore to God. Resist the devil, and he will flee from you.

Eph 6:14–18 (TCNT,KJV) Stand your ground, then, with Truth for your belt, and with righteousness for your breastplate, and with the readiness to serve the Good News of Peace as shoes for your feet. At every onslaught take up faith for your shield; for with it you will be able to extinguish all the flaming darts of the evil one. (Above all, taking the shield of faith, wherewith you shall be able to quench all the fiery darts of the wicked. Take the helmet of salvation, and the sword of the Spirit, which is the Word of God.) Pray in Spirit at all times. Be intent upon this, with unwearying perseverance and supplication for all Christ's people.

Col 2:15a (AMP) [God] disarmed the principalities and powers that were ranged against us and made a bold display and public example of them.

Col 2:15a (WNT) And the hostile princes and rulers He stripped off from Himself, and boldly displayed them as His conquests.

Ph 2:9–11 (KJV) God also hath highly exalted Him, and given Him a Name which is above every name. That at the Name of Jesus every knee should bow, of things (of beings) in heaven, and things in earth, and things under the earth; and that every tongue should confess that Jesus Christ is Lord, to the glory of God the Father.

Eph 1:22,23 (KJV) (God) hath put all things under His feet, and gave Him to be the head over all things to the church, which is His body, the fulness of Him that filleth all in all.

Eph 1:22–2:2 (AMP) And He has put all things under His feet and has appointed Him the universal and supreme Head of the church [a headship exercised throughout the church], which is His body, the fullness of Him Who fills all in all [for in that body lives the full measure of Him Who makes everything complete, and Who fills everything everywhere with Himself]. And you [He made alive], when you were dead (slain) by [your] trespasses and sins in which at one time you walked [habitually]. You were following the course and fashion of this world [were under the sway of the tendency of this present age], following the prince of the power of the air. [You were obedient to and under the control of] the [demon] spirit that still constantly works in the sons of disobedience [the careless, the rebellious, and the unbelieving, who go against the purposes of God].

Eph 5:30 (KJV) We are members of His body, of His flesh, and of His bones.

1Co 6:20 (KJV) Ye are bought with a price: therefore glorify God in your body, and in your spirit, which are God's.

1Jn 4:4b (KJV) Greater is He that is in you, than he that is in the world.

Is 54:17a (KJV) No weapon that is formed against thee shall prosper.

Lk 10:19 (KJV) Behold, I give unto you power to tread on serpents and scorpions, and over all the power of the enemy: and nothing shall by any means hurt you.

Mt 18:18,19 (KJV) Verily I say unto you, Whatsoever ye shall bind on earth shall be bound in heaven: and whatsoever ye shall loose on earth shall be loosed in heaven. Again I say unto you, That if two of you shall agree on earth as touching anything that they shall ask, it shall be done for them of My Father which is in heaven.

Mt 18:18,19 (AMP) Truly I tell you, whatever you forbid and declare to be improper and unlawful on earth must be what is already forbidden in heaven, and whatever you permit and declare proper and lawful on earth must be what is already permitted in heaven. Again I tell you, if two of you on earth agree (harmonize together, make a symphony together) about whatever [anything and everything] they may ask, it will come to pass and be done for them by My Father in heaven.

Ro 8:31b,32 (NIV) If God is for us, who can be against us? He who did not spare his own Son, but gave him up for us all—how will he not also, along with him, graciously give us all things?

Lk 17:5,6 (WNT) And the Apostles said to the Lord, "Give us faith." "If your faith," replied the Lord, "is like a mustard seed, you might command this black–mulberry–tree, 'Tear up your roots and plant yourself in the sea,' and instantly it would obey you."

Lk 4:39 (KJV) And He stood over her, and rebuked the fever; and it left her: and immediately she arose and ministered unto them.

Lk 4:39 (GW) He bent over her, ordered the fever to leave, and it went away. She got up immediately and prepared a meal for them.

Lk 4:39 He spoke and rebuked the fever, commanding it to leave her body, and it left.
(Rebuke your illness and command it to leave in the name of Jesus.)

Lk 17:5,6 (NAB) And the apostles said to the Lord, "Increase our faith." The Lord replied, "If you have faith the size of a mustard seed, you would say to [this] mulberry tree, 'Be uprooted and planted in the sea,' and it would obey you.

Mk 11:22–23 Jesus answered them "Have faith in
God; take hold on God's faithfulness. For I assure
you whoever says to this mountain, 'Move! Be
removed and be cast into the sea!' and shall not
doubt in his heart, does not waver, but believes
that what he says will come to pass, he shall have
whatever he says. It shall be granted him."

Mt 17:20 (KJV) And Jesus said unto them, Because
of your unbelief: for verily I say unto you, If ye
have faith as a grain of mustard seed, ye shall say
unto this mountain, Remove hence to yonder
place; and it shall remove; and nothing shall be
impossible unto you.

Mt 17:20 (DBY) And He (Jesus) says to them,
Because of your unbelief; for verily I say unto you,
If you have faith as a grain of mustard seed, you
shall say to this mountain, Be transported hence
there, and it shall transport itself; and nothing
shall be impossible to you.

Mt 19:26b, Mk 10:27b (KJV) With God ALL things
are possible.

He 11:1 (KJV) Now faith is the substance of things hoped for, the evidence of things not seen.

Ro 10:17 (KJV) Faith comes by hearing, and hearing by the Word of God.

2Co 5:7 (KJV) For we walk by faith, not by sight.

2Co 5:7 We guide ourselves by faith, not by what we see; not by external appearance.

Eph 3:12 (AMP) In whom, because of our faith in Him, we dare to have the boldness (courage and confidence) of free access (an unreserved approach to God with freedom and without fear).

He 10:23 (GW) We must continue to hold firmly to our declaration of faith. The one who made the promise is faithful.

2Co 1:20a All the promises of God are Yes and Amen.

He 10:35,36 (AMP) Do not, therefore, fling away your fearless confidence, for it carries a great and glorious compensation of reward. For you have need of steadfast patience and endurance, so that you may perform and fully accomplish the will of God, and thus receive and carry away [and enjoy to the full] what is promised.

Ph 2:13 (WNT) It is God Himself Whose power creates within you both the desire and the power to execute His gracious will.

Ga 5:6b (KJV) Faith which worketh by love.

1Jn 2:5 (AMP) But he who keeps (treasures) His Word [who bears in mind His precepts, who observes His message in its entirety], truly in him has the love of and for God been perfected (completed, reached maturity). By this we may perceive (know, recognize, and be sure) that we are in Him.

Eph 3:17–21 (KJV) That Christ may dwell in your hearts by faith; that ye, being rooted and grounded in love, may be able to comprehend with all saints what is the breadth, and length, and depth, and height; and to know the love of Christ, which passeth knowledge, that ye might be filled with all the fulness of God. Now unto Him that is able to do exceeding abundantly above all that we ask or think, according to the power that worketh in us, unto Him be glory in the church by Christ Jesus throughout all ages, world without end. Amen.

Eph 3:17–21 (AMP) May Christ through your faith [actually] dwell (settle down, abide, make His permanent home) in your hearts! May you be rooted deep in love and founded securely on love, that you may have the power and be strong to apprehend and grasp with all the saints [God's devoted people, the experience of that love] what is the breadth and length and height and depth [of it]; [that you may really come] to know [practically, through experience for yourselves] the love of Christ, which far surpasses mere knowledge [without experience]; that you may be filled [through all your being] unto all the fullness of God [may have the richest measure of the divine Presence, and become a body wholly filled and flooded with God Himself]! Now to Him Who, by (in consequence of) the [action of His] power that is at work within us, is able to [carry out His purpose and] do superabundantly, far over and above all that we [dare] ask or think [infinitely beyond our highest prayers, desires, thoughts, hopes, or dreams]—to Him be glory in the church and in Christ Jesus throughout all generations forever and ever. Amen (so be it).

Eph 4:15a (KJV) Speaking the Truth in love, may grow up into Him in all things.

Eph 4:29 (WNT) Let no unwholesome words ever pass your lips, but let all your words be good for benefiting others according to the need of the moment, so that they may be a means of blessing to the hearers.

Pr 15:26b (KJV) The words of the pure are pleasant words.

Pr 16:24 (KJV) Pleasant words are as an honeycomb, sweet to the soul, and health to the bones.

Pr 21:23 (KJV) Whoso keepeth his mouth and his tongue keepeth his soul from troubles.

Pr 16:23 (KJV) The heart of the wise teacheth his mouth, and addeth learning to his lips.

Pr 12:18b (KJV) The tongue of the wise is health.

Pr 12:18b (NASB) The tongue of the wise brings healing.

Pr 13:2a (NASB) From the fruit of a man's mouth he enjoys good.

Ps 103:5 (KJV) Who satisfieth thy mouth with good things; so that thy youth is renewed like the eagle's.

Pr 18:20 (KJV) A man's belly shall be satisfied with the fruit of his mouth; and with the increase of his lips shall he be filled.

Pr 8:6 (KJV) Hear; for I will speak of excellent things; and the opening of My lips shall be right things.

Ps 119:172 (DBY) My tongue shall speak aloud of Thy Word; for all Thy commandments are righteousness.

Re 12:11a (KJV) They overcame him by the Blood of the Lamb, and by the word of their testimony.
(We overcome satan by professing what the Word says the Blood does in ALL its aspects.)

Mt 12:37 (KJV) For by thy words thou shalt be justified, and by thy words thou shalt be condemned.

Pr 18:21 (KJV) Death and life are in the power of the tongue: and they that love it shall eat the fruit thereof.

Pr 6:2 (KJV) Thou art snared with the words of thy mouth, thou art taken with the words of thy mouth.

Pr 12:13,14a (AMP) The wicked is [dangerously] snared by the transgression of his lips, but the [uncompromisingly] righteous shall come out of trouble. From the fruit of his words a man shall be satisfied with good.

Ps 39:1a (KJV) I said, I will take heed to my ways, that I sin not with my tongue: I will keep my mouth with a bridle.

Ps 50:23 (KJV) Whoso offereth praise glorifieth Me: and to him that ordereth his conversation aright will I show the salvation of God.

Ps 56:10 (KJV) In God will I praise His Word: in the Lord will I praise His Word.

Ps 119:175 (KJV) Let my soul live, and it shall praise Thee; and let Thy judgments help me.

Ps 119:164a (KJV) Seven times a day do I praise Thee.

Ps 118:1 (KJV) O give thanks unto the Lord; for He is good: because His mercy endureth forever.

Ps 71:6b (KJV) My praise shall be continually of Thee.

2Ch 20:21b (KJV) Praise the Lord; for His mercy endureth forever.

Ps 57:7 (KJV) My heart is fixed, O God, my heart is fixed: I will sing and give praise.

Eph 5:19 (KJV) Speaking to yourselves in psalms and hymns and spiritual songs, singing and making melody in your heart to the Lord.

Col 3:16 (KJV) Let the Word of Christ dwell in you richly in all wisdom; teaching and admonishing one another in psalms and hymns and spiritual songs, singing with grace in your hearts to the Lord.

Ph 4:8 (KJV) Finally, brethren, whatsoever things are true, whatsoever things are honest, whatsoever things are just, whatsoever things are pure, whatsoever things are lovely, whatsoever things are of good report; if there be any virtue, and if there be any praise, think (meditate) on these things.

2Co 9:8 (KJV) God is able to make all grace abound toward you; that you, always having ALL sufficiency in ALL things, may abound to every good work.

2Co 2:14a Thanks be to God, Who ALWAYS causes us to triumph in Messiah.

1Pt 2:24b By Jesus' stripes I am healed.

Ro 4:17b (AKJV) God calls those things which be not as though they were.

(I call those things which be not as though they are.)

1Pt 4:11a If I speak, let me speak as the Oracles of God.

Is 55:11 (LEB) So shall be my word that goes out from my mouth. It shall not return to me without success, but shall accomplish what I desire and be successful in the thing for which I sent it.

Ps 107:20 Thank You Lord, that You sent Your Word and healed me!

Ps 118:17 (KJV) I shall not die, but live, and declare the works of the Lord.

Ps 118:17 (GW) I will not die, but I will live and tell what the Lord has done.

Faith Action

An additional step towards the goal of
your faith!

Now for a little extra boost. When a contractor begins a building, he goes forth knowing he has the correct tools and that they will all work properly to accomplish what he has set out to do. He looks at the blueprints to see what the building will look like. All along, as he is working toward the finished building, he sees it in his mind through the blueprints. Your God–given imagination can work much the same way. I suggest you go find a number of pictures of yourself where you are looking good, healthy, and strong; the way you desire to be. Use these to help you

> The Word is the true blueprint. He is the life-giving Spirit. He gives life to the Word in you.

keep the finished product of your faith in the forefront of your mind. Put them in places where you will see them several times a day. Look on them upon arising and let them be the last thing you see before bed. Also, choose some Scriptures and personalize them. For example: Isaiah 53:5, "With His stripes *I* am healed," and Psalms 107:20, "He sent His Word and healed *me* ..." Better still: "With *Your* stripes *I* am healed," and "*You* sent *Your* Word and healed *me* ..." Select the ones that are the most powerful and faith–building for you, and write them out on little notes and place them with the pictures.

By the way, the definition of vigor is: "1. active strength of body: good physical condition 2. mental energy 3. strength or force in general; powerful action; potency."

Choose verses that will cause you to see yourself the way you want to be—the way God sees you. He already sees the finished product. He sees you with abundant life, health, strength, power, vitality, ability, anointing; energized, full of vim and vigor. Remember to read the words aloud as this will intensify the faith power fourfold: as you *see* the pictures, *see* the words, *speak* the words, and *hear* the words.

Here are some other positive words that you can claim for yourself.

Thank you Lord that I am (have):

> *active*
> *energetic*
> *robust*
> *thriving*
> *motivated*
> *determined*
> *productive*
> *industrious*
> *hardworking*
> *creative*
> *excellent memory*
> *restored*
> *flourishing*
> *regenerated*
> *rejuvenated*
> *resurrection life*

Destiny Arise

Expectation!

Believe there is life in God's Words. All the life that you need is in these Words. If you will work daily to plant them in your heart, tending them properly by watering (speaking and meditating on them) and weeding (removing any hindrances), the Holy Spirit will cause them to produce that life, and all it contains, *in* you.

You *can* be well; you *can* walk in divine health. It *is* God's destiny for you. Reach for it with all your might and don't stop until healing arises! That desire for health in your heart is your spirit's yearning to be conformed to His image; to show forth His glory in the earth; to walk in His resurrection life.

Make this your greatest objective, your highest aspiration, your unalterable purpose for living:

I SHALL NOT DIE, BUT LIVE, AND DECLARE THE WONDERFUL WORKS OF THE LORD!

Healing arise!